YOUR KNOWLEDGE HAS VALUE

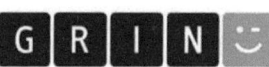

Gary Elliott

Adolescent Schizophrenia. The background

GRIN Verlag

Bibliografische Information der Deutschen Nationalbibliothek:

Die Deutsche Bibliothek verzeichnet diese Publikation in der Deutschen National-
bibliografie; detaillierte bibliografische Daten sind im Internet über http://dnb.d-
nb.de/ abrufbar.

Imprint:

Copyright © 2010 GRIN Verlag GmbH
Druck und Bindung: Books on Demand GmbH, Norderstedt Germany
ISBN: 978-3-656-68023-9

This book at GRIN:

http://www.grin.com/en/e-book/275087/adolescent-schizophrenia-the-background

GARY WILLIAM ELLIOTT

CURRICULUM DESIGN COURSE

ADOLESCENT SCHIZOPHRENIA

ATLANTIC INTERNATIONAL UNIVERSITY
HONOLULU, HAWAII
December 2010

TABLE OF CONTENTS

1. Schizophrenia – the background

1.1 Introduction and Definitions

Adolescent schizophrenia is a largely misunderstood, under-studied area of schizophrenia. Adolescence is a period of development marked at the beginning by the onset of puberty and at the end by the attainment of physiological or psychological maturity (Dictionary of Psychology). Schizophrenia may be defined as a general label for a number of psychotic disorders with various cognitive, emotional and behavioural manifestations and is a term that originated with Eugen Bleuler in 1911 as a replacement for the term Dementia Praecox.

The above definition may seem a little too academic, but the term literally refers to a 'splitting in the mind'; a dissociation between emotions and cognition. Schizophrenia is a severe brain disease that results in a person losing touch with reality. The disease is accompanied by hallucinations, delusions, disorganized speech and behaviour, among others. These are just a few of the accompanying symptoms but together they affect social interactions and thought processes and have serious impact on the functioning of the sufferer.

We do not know exactly what causes schizophrenia, but it affects 1 in 100 people and is one of the most serious mental disorders (Furnham, 2008). The lifetime prevalence of schizophrenia in the United States of America is about 1 percent. The age of onset for schizophrenia occurs earlier in males than females, with the age group 16-25 years of age having the highest prevalence rates (Castle & Murray, 1993). Although the disease usually appears in late adolescence or early adulthood, seemingly without warning, it is a gradual disease that develops over many years (Gur & Johnson, 2006). Schizophrenia is very rare before age 11 but symptoms can appear as early as the mid- to late teens and are usually seen before age twenty; with most cases developing between age fifteen and twenty-five (Haycock, 2009). As such, a diagnosis is seldom made before age 18 (early-onset schizophrenia) and after age 50.

While the symptoms of schizophrenia may cause psychotic behaviour, most are not particularly violent and will not strike out at other. As little as 4% of violent acts are committed by people with schizophrenia and homicides by those who suffer with the disease is approximately 1 in 3000 cases. We admittedly still know very little about schizophrenia and are unable to prevent its occurrence but with early detection and intervention the sufferer can have a better quality of life.

1.2 History of Schizophrenia

It is agreed that we do not know how long schizophrenia has been around but mental illnesses have evidence in tablets, carvings and writings of the ancient world. While these inscriptions give a hint of its existence, they are too vague to give recognition for the symptoms and features of schizophrenia.

A number of researchers will concede that schizophrenia may have been around in the late Middle Ages. In the sixteenth century, Shakespeare's plays acknowledge mental illness but Torrey believes that the first 'true' description of schizophrenia only materialized in the early nineteenth century.

As early as 1809, a superintendent of a British hospital, John Haslam, outlined a description of the symptoms of schizophrenia in *Observations on Madness and Melancholy*. During the course of 1801-1809, a French physician, Philippe Pinel described many cases of schizophrenia in his patients. In 1834, a Russian author Nikolai Gogol provided an early, yet complete description of schizophrenia in his short story *Diary of a Madman*. A French psychiatrist, Benedict-Augustin Morel, coined the Latin term *dementia praecox* (1852) which meant early or premature loss of mind to describe schizophrenia. Paranoid psychosis was first described in 1868; disorganized schizophrenia in 1869 and catatonic schizophrenia in 1872. In 1896, Emil Kraepelin unified the distinct categories of schizophrenia (hebephrenic, catatonic and paranoid) under the name *dementia praecox*.

In the twentieth century, Eugen Bleuler (1911), replaced Kraepelin's term of 'dementia praecox' with 'schizophrenia'. The choice of term was focused on the thought processes rather than on the outcome of the illness. Bleuler realized that the disease caused a 'splitting of the mind' from the reality around them. This splitting of the mind caused the misconception of a split personality. Bleuler believed that schizophrenia consisted of more than one disease and the disease could be traced to damage to specific areas of the brain.

Early theorists proposed that psychopathology (especially schizophrenia) was the result of inconsistency in family communications (Bateson, Jackson, Haley, & Weakland, 1956). In recent years, biological factors have been associated with depression, suicide and certain forms of schizophrenia (Sue, Sue & Sue, 1997). The specifics of causal factors in the development of schizophrenia will be discussed in detail later in this paper.

1.3 Early Treatment

Although schizophrenia as a disorder materialized in the nineteenth and early twentieth century, doctors were unable to treat it. Three early methods of treatment are discussed below:

Insulin Coma Therapy was developed by a Polish psychiatrist and neurophysiologist Manfred Joshua Sakel in the 1930s. Inducing an insulin coma in his patients, he discovered that the lowering of the blood sugar levels depleted the brain and body of energy. Deprived of energy, the brain shuts down, causing convulsions and eventually coma. Sakel saw improvement in the symptoms of his patients with schizophrenia in 90% of cases. Eventually, other doctors in the field discovered that this form of therapy had little effect in the long term and it was discontinued when tranquilizer type drugs entered the market.

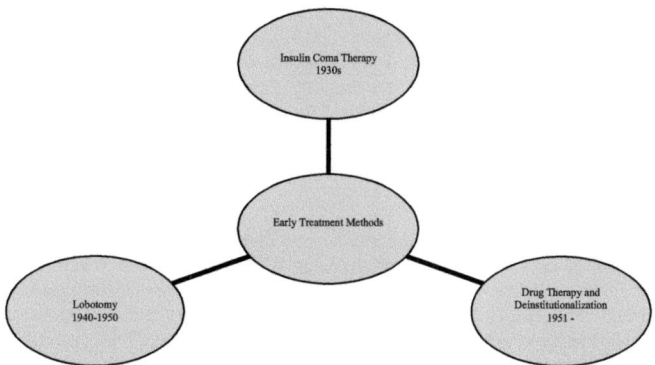

Lobotomy as a procedure for the elimination of schizophrenia was popularized in the 1940s and early 1950s by the neurologist Walter Freeman. This psychosurgical procedure was pioneered by Moniz and Lima; it involved the cutting of the nerve connections between the area of the brain above the eye (the prefrontal cortex) and the rest of the brain. Freeman used an ice pick-like instrument in his variation of the lobotomy (the transorbital lobotomy) that simplified the procedure. The ice pick pierced the thin bone behind the eye socket and was pushed into the brain; back and forth movements severed the connections. Although this was a fast procedure (lasting only a few minutes) it was a medical fad. A staggering 18 000 lobotomies were conducted in the US alone before doctors realized that it did more harm than good. Although psychotic patients were pacified, it left them apathetic, emotionally stunted and unable to concentrate. In effect, the lobotomy caused severe brain damage to the patient and was discontinued in 1951.

Drug therapy and deinstitutionalization began with the introduction of antipsychotic and other mental health medication. In 1955, state mental institutions in the US housed approximately 560 000 patients; by the year 2000 this number has dropped by some 90%. The introduction of drug therapy and public policy has produced an improvement in the understanding of schizophrenia and thus a decline in long-term hospitalization of patients. In 1951, French psychiatrists Jean Delay and Pierre Deniker discovered that chlorpromazine (Thorazine) was extremely effective in treating schizophrenia (Sue, Sue & Sue, 1997). In addition, the Community Health Act of 1963 assisted in the move to rehabilitate patients and deinstitutionalize them (Haycock, 2009).

2. Causes of Schizophrenia

While we acknowledge that relatively little is known about the causes of schizophrenia, current research into the disease focuses on brain abnormalities, genetics and environment factors (Gur & Johnson, 2006). The disease may have a viral cause but is most certainly precipitated by stress.

2.1 Brain Abnormalities

The most accepted hypothesis among researchers is that schizophrenia is a brain disease. A reduction in metabolic activity in the frontal cortex of people who have been diagnosed with schizophrenia has been noted. The central nervous system uses neurotransmitters to carry information in chemical form across the synapse. Injury to the brain and disease can disrupt the process by which neurons send messages to one another. The neurotransmitter dopamine has been associated with schizophrenia, although serotonin, glutamate and others may be impaired in different brain regions of the limbic structures, ganglia, prefrontal cortex, temporal lobes and the cerebellum (Haycock, 2009). Tyrosine hydroxylase, a chemical related to dopamine has been found in large quantities in schizophrenics, implying that excess tyrosine may create an excess of dopamine. There are a number of different dopaminergic receptors that are metabotropic, with D_1 and D_2 receptors having a direct link to schizophrenia. In addition, a higher level of norepinephrine has been found in the brain of schizophrenics, and some researchers suspect that an excess of serotonin may be present in the brain (Gur & Johnson, 2006).

Banich (2004) notes that both microsomatagnosia (the sensation that parts of the body are too big) and macrosomatagmosia (the sensation that parts of the body are too small) can occur with schizophrenics. Schizophrenia has been associated with temporal lobe dysfunction, as the temporal lobe aids in creating a mental map of the body. These temporal regions dysfunction has been associated with the delusions that schizophrenics experience.

While an excess of dopamine has been implicated in the development of schizophrenia (Cooper, Bloom & Roth, 1986), some believe that schizophrenia can 'cause' the secretion of excess amounts of dopamine. It is important to note also that other researchers believe that there is no biological marker for schizophrenia at all (Szymanski, Kane & Lieberman, 1991). However, in contradiction, it is estimated that anywhere from 20 to 65 percent of schizophrenics show some sign of neurological abnormalities (Buchsbaum, 1990).

2.2 Genetics

Is there any evidence that schizophrenia runs in families? Since 1980, 11 major family studies have shown that the risk for schizophrenia in first-degree relatives is higher than the general population (Gur & Johnson, 2006). Parents, siblings and children of schizophrenics are twelve times more likely (5.9%) to develop the disease than the general population. Biological relatives and depressed adoptees are more likely to share the same disorder than adopted relatives (Loehln, Willerman & Horn, 1988).

Heredity does seem to play some role in schizophrenia, concordance and adoption research suggests that the tendency for schizophrenia to run in families is partly due to genetic factors, with a concordance rate of 50% for identical twins and only around 18% for fraternal twins (Berk, 2000). In addition, relatives of individuals with schizophrenia are more likely to have paranoid personality disorder than people who do not have a relative with schizophrenia (Barlow & Durand, 2005).

While a specific gene that causes schizophrenia has not been identified, it is agreed that there is something in the genetic make-up of a person that predisposes him to schizophrenia. People with schizophrenia tend to have a missing section of DNA on chromosome 1, two missing sections on chromosome 15 and a missing section on chromosome 22. The National Institute of Mental Health estimates that 60% of the factors that cause schizophrenia are related to a genetic susceptibility (Haycock, 2009).

2.3 Environment

It has been suggested that stress-inducing factors in the environment promote schizophrenia in individuals who are susceptible. These triggers may include the following:

- Nutrition
- Viruses and parasites
- Maternal stress
- Maternal viral infection during pregnancy

- Advanced parental age
- Development problems before birth
- Complications during birth
- Environmental toxins

(Haycock, 2009)

A parasite called toxoplasma gondii may be responsible for schizophrenia in some cases. This protozoa is found in undercooked meat and cat faeces. Haloperidol is an antipsychotic drug that targets the protozoan, and may be used in eradicating the parasite. Although there is no specific schizophrenia virus, it is agreed that a virus or viruses can contribute to the development of the disease.

Barlow & Durand (2005) suggest that whether one lives in a city or the country may be associated with the risk of developing schizophrenia. It is interesting to note that the incidence of schizophrenia in males living in the city is 38% higher that their counterparts living in the country. This idea of increased stress levels being a precipitating factor in the development of schizophrenia is supported by the tenets of Haycock (2009), who suggests that stress to a pregnant mother during the first six months of pregnancy produces an increased risk of giving birth to a child that will develop schizophrenia later in his life.

3. Schizophrenia Types

The classification of schizophrenia remains complex because of the diversity of symptoms. These symptoms include; delusions, hallucinations, disorganized speech (incoherence, loose association, use of nonsense words), disorganized behaviour (dress, body posture, personal hygiene), negative and flat emotions, poor insight into their problems and depression (Furnham, 2008). Symptoms of schizophrenia and the diagnostic criteria will be discussed later, but adding to the complex nature of categorizing schizophrenia is the recognition of five types of schizophrenic disorders. While they have different characteristics there is little difference has been found in their response to treatment (Lieberman, 1995).

The categories of schizophrenia are given diagrammatically below and will be discussed individually thereafter.

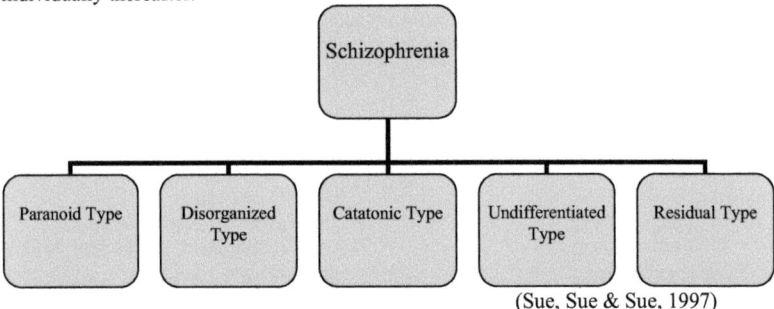

(Sue, Sue & Sue, 1997)

3.1 Paranoid Schizophrenia

This is the most common type and is characterized by delusions or auditory hallucinations and the absence of such symptoms as disorganized speech and behaviour or flat affect. The deluded individual believes that other people are plotting against them, talking behind their back or are aiming to harm them in some way. They will be constantly suspicious of others and their motives. Paranoid schizophrenics have delusions of control, grandeur and persecution. These individuals are often prone to outbursts of anger particularly when they feel that they are being persecuted (Sue, Sue & Sue, 1997).

3.2 Disorganized Schizophrenia

This category includes the most psychotic and difficult to treat patients. It was formerly known as hebephrenic schizophrenia, and appears at a younger age than paranoid schizophrenia. These patients tend to have poor hygiene with an unkempt appearance. This category sees the patient's condition deteriorating rapidly without treatment. Disorganized speech will be present and speech is often interspersed with laughter or silliness. They manifest bizarre thoughts and language, with sudden inappropriate emotional outbursts. There is a severe decline in routine behaviour and grooming and

8

bathing suffers. Patients may have delusions and/or hallucinations but they are not as elaborate or organized as those displayed in paranoid schizophrenia (Haycock, 2009).

3.3 Catatonic Schizophrenia

'Catatonic' comes from the Greek 'to stretch or draw tight'. This type of schizophrenia is marked by either extreme excitement or complete immobility. Symptoms of this sub-type include excessive, purposeless activity, extreme negativism or physical resistance, peculiar movement, echolalia (repetition of other's words) or echopraxia (repetition of other's movements). Catatonics may talk and shout constantly, or run until they fall from exhaustion. They do have a tendency to be violent but the disorder is extremely rare.

Sufferers of excited catatonia are hyperactive and agitated, while people with withdrawn catatonia are unresponsive for prolonged periods of time, adopting strange postures and refusing to move (Sue, Sue & Sue, 1997).

3.4 Undifferentiated Schizophrenia

Undifferentiated schizophrenia is only diagnosed when the symptoms of the patient cannot be laced into one of the above categories. Although the patient may not have symptoms of paranoia, disorganization or catatonia, they do display symptoms of delusions, hallucinations disorganized speech or behaviour or 'negative' symptoms (these will be discussed later).

3.5 Residual Schizophrenia

This category describes those patients who do not fall into a classification of paranoid, disorganized, catatonic or undifferentiated. There are sufficient 'negative' symptoms such as social withdrawal, reduced or limited emotional range, and lack of ambition for large and small projects, and reluctance to speak, in order to register as not fully recovered from the previously existing symptoms of schizophrenia. It is common to see residual schizophrenics display fleeting hallucinations but they are not as severe, disorganized or persistent (Haycock, 2009).

4. Symptoms

There is no one symptom that characterizes schizophrenia and a diagnosis of schizophrenia involves the presence of several symptoms that have been present for months. Schizophrenia is described by Gur & Johnson (2006) as a disorder of perception; the idea that reality to other people is not 'real' to the person with schizophrenia and unfortunately the schizophrenic is not aware that his perception of what is 'real' is actually not. The American Psychiatric Association divides the symptoms of schizophrenia into two broad categories; those of positive symptoms and negative symptoms. Positive symptoms are active manifestations of abnormal behaviour, or an excess or distortion of normal behaviour and include delusions and hallucinations. Negative symptoms involve deficits in normal behaviour on such dimensions as affect, speech and motivation. Disorganized symptoms include rambling speech, erratic behaviour and inappropriate affect (Barlow & Durand, 2005).

As noted in the previous section, schizophrenia is classified into five types, each with its own specific symptoms but typically, the schizophrenic shows a combination of symptoms from eight categories.

Symptom Categories in Schizophrenia

Category	Symptom(s)
Content of thought	A delusion or false belief.
Form of thought	A formal thought disorder involving abnormalities in the way a person's thought processes are organized. "Loose association" in which ideas shift from one unrelated topic to another, is a common example of this type of symptom.
Perception	Hallucinations or the reporting of experiences for which no observable eliciting stimuli appear to exist.
Affect	Disturbed emotions. Most common are emotions that are blunted, flat, or inappropriate to the situation.
Sense of self	Confusion about self-identity. The person may feel unreal or controlled by outside forces.
Volition	Reduced motivation and interest in pursuing almost any sort of goal. These symptoms interfere severely with a person's ability to work.
Relationship to the external world	Withdrawal from the external world and preoccupation with internal fantasies and odd ideas. These symptoms are sometimes called autistic.
Psychomotor behaviour	Abnormalities of movement, including rocking, pacing, stereotyped actions, and bizarre behavioural rituals. Some patients diagnosed with schizophrenia become almost totally immobile; others take on a disheveled look or dress oddly, against social norms.

(Banich, 2004)

4.1 Positive Symptoms

Positive symptoms are not positive in the sense of being affirmative, they are positive in the sense of existing or being present as opposed to being absent or deficient. In simpler terms, positive symptoms are additions to normal functioning. The 'additions' distort the hearing, speech or thoughts of the schizophrenic. Positive symptoms include:

- Delusions
- Hallucinations
- Disorganized thought and speech

Delusions – there are nine types of delusions observed in schizophrenics. Delusions of grandeur; believing that they have been assigned by God, who has given them

10

supernatural powers to fulfill a specific task. Thought control; they believe that an external force is planting thoughts into their mind. Passivity; they believe that they are under the control of an external force. Reference; they believe that they are always the centre of attention, that others are construing behind their back. Poverty; he may believe that he has no money or security even though evidence indicates the opposite. Persecution; they believe that they are the subject of elaborate plots against them. Guilt; they are often convinced that they have done something unforgivable. Sickness; he may be convinced that he has a terrible disease even though he is physically healthy. Jealousy; a belief that his wife or significant other has been unfaithful even without evidence (Haycock, 2009).

Hallucinations can be defined as sensory events that are not based on any specific external event. The schizophrenic may hear voices or see people who have already died; these voices are referred to as auditory hallucinations.

Disorganized speech includes the schizophrenic jumping from one topic to another, not answering direct questions or going off on a tangent, essentially talking illogically. Occasionally the schizophrenic talks in words and sentences that are completely unintelligible.

4.2 Negative Symptoms

Negative symptoms represent characteristic behaviour that seems to be removed by the disease. There is a gradual withdrawal from the world, from one's family and from oneself.

Alogia refers to difficulty in communicating; this results in a reduction in speech.
Affective flattening or blunted affect refers to a lack of emotional expression.
Avolition is the inability to initiate plans of action or to motivate oneself.
Anhedonia is the inability to enjoy activities that were previously enjoyed.

It is these negative symptoms that cause the most difficulty for the family of schizophrenics and cause the most disruption to daily functioning. The schizophrenic typically is quite oblivious to what is happening around them and display indifference towards people and events occurring around him.

4.3 Gender

There are differences in how schizophrenia affects the sexes. There is currently speculation as to the reason for this difference and conflicting ideas focus on hormonal differences in the brain and the course of the disease during the years of puberty. It is however, agreed that schizophrenia occurs earlier in males than in females, with ages 16-25 having the highest prevalence rates (Castle & Murray, 1993). In addition, males tend to develop the symptoms of schizophrenia an average of three to four years earlier than females (Gur & Johnson, 2006).

The median age for onset of schizophrenia for males is the early twenties, implying that first signs of the disease occur at around the age of twenty-three on average but may, and do, occur earlier in some cases. Although females tend to develop the disease later than males, they have a more rapid decline into schizophrenia than their male counterparts. If schizophrenia occurs after age forty (late onset), it is more prevalent in females.

4.4 Suicide

It is estimated that approximately 40% of schizophrenia patients will attempt suicide (National Alliance for Research on Schizophrenia and Depression). The Schizophrenia Society of Canada places this figure slightly higher at 50%. Completed suicides claim an approximate 10 to 15% of sufferers, which is a higher prevalence rate than the general population. As such, suicide is the primary cause of premature death in schizophrenics.

As the patient struggles with the disease they are often subject to severe depression, losing hope that they will ever recover from this disease. Males are at a higher risk for severe depression and thus constitute the greatest percentage of suicide attempts.

Who Is at Risk for Suicide?

+ People who have tried it before
+ People who have talked about it before
+ People who are anxious, depressed and exhausted
+ People with ready access to lethal weapons and toxic substances
+ People who have talked about wanting to die
+ People who have all of a sudden prepared a will or given away their possessions
+ People who are in mourning or facing a crisis
+ People who act and seem as if they think things are hopeless
+ People with a family history of suicide

(Gur & Johnson, 2006)

5. Warning Signs

The symptoms of schizophrenia are numerous and the disease causes severe disruption to social, occupational and recreational functioning. As such, it is imperative that the disease is identified as early as possible and intervention on an ongoing basis can assist in allowing schizophrenics to live functional lives and improve significantly. A good prognosis is supported by late onset of the disease, a good family support system, higher IQs and a strong social and vocational history (Gur & Johnson, 2006).

Early symptoms of the disease, known as 'prodromal' symptoms may begin to manifest two to six years prior to the first psychotic episode. These, often subtle signs include:
• Reduced concentration and attention
• Decreased motivation and energy
• Mood changes, such as depression and anxiety
• Sleep difficulties

- Social withdrawal
- Suspiciousness
- Irritability
- Neglected physical appearance
- Decline in academic performance and abandonment of previous interests

(Gur & Johnson, 2006)

5.1 In Early Childhood

Although there seems to be little distinction between the pathology of schizophrenia in adolescence and adulthood, there is a difference in the severity of the symptoms. If the disease begins early, the patient tends to display more severe brain abnormalities, more abnormalities in brain cells, poorer future outcome and a greater genetic burden based on their relatives who have or had psychiatric illnesses. Children tend to be less social and more emotionally distant than other children their age. It is common to see a marked decline in the intellectual or thinking ability of the child. This manifests as a drastic decline in understanding, reading, writing or thinking. There is usually also serious problems with schooling, particularly low scores on tests, this is due to cognitive problems that causes difficulty with memory, concentration, attendance, self-discipline, organizational ability and social skills (Haycock, 2009).

5.2 In Adolescence

In most cases, the presence of schizophrenia does not become evident until well into the adolescent years; unfortunately the cause for this accelerated appearance of the disease is still unknown. Some indicators of the disease in adolescence might include seeing things or hearing voices that are not seen or heard by other people, the display of odd or eccentric behaviour and speech, unusual or bizarre thoughts, the confusing of TV or dreams with real life, regressive child-like behaviour and severe anxiety and fearfulness.

5.3 Prevention

It is still not possible to prevent schizophrenia, but with early intervention we are able to reduce the negative impact of the disease on the patient. The critical aspect is early identification; this can be achieved by identifying risk factors for the disease. Some critical risk factors for the development of schizophrenia include family history, having older parents, maternal infections or complications during pregnancy, social adjustment problems during childhood and adolescence and velo-cardio-facial syndrome (American Journal of Preventive Medicine, Feb 2004).

Adolescents with a family history of schizophrenia can lower their risk by not using illegal drugs or abusing alcohol. If a predisposition exists, they may be susceptible to bad reactions to recreational drugs. Street drugs such as marijuana, cocaine, hallucinogens and methamphetamines can precipitate the onset of schizophrenia (Haycock, 2009).

6. Diagnosing Schizophrenia

Adolescence is a time of life in which instability and uncertainty are often present in the personality of even the well-adjusted child. The difficulty associated with a diagnosis of schizophrenia in teenagers can be compounded as a result of substance abuse, conduct disorder or attention deficit/hyperactivity disorder (ADHD); alternatively the teenager can have all of these disorders at the same time.

Schizophrenia is a disturbance lasting at least six months and including a mixture of at least one month of two or more of the following symptoms: delusions, hallucinations, disorganized speech, grossly disorganized or catatonic behaviour and negative symptoms (Gur & Johnson, 2006).

The teenager should have a complete physical examination, including blood and urine analysis for the presence of commonly abused drugs and other medical conditions. A psychiatrist will use the Diagnostic and Statistical Manual of Mental Disorders to accurately diagnose schizophrenia in the teen. The DSM-IV outlines the Criteria for Schizophrenia as follows:

A. At least two of the following symptoms lasting for at least one month in the active phase (exception: only one symptom if it involves bizarre delusions or if hallucinations involve running commentary on the person or two or more voices talking with each other).
   a. Delusions
   b. Hallucinations
   c. Disorganized speech (incoherence or frequent derailment)
   d. Grossly disorganized or catatonic behaviour
   e. Negative symptoms (flat affect, avolition, alogia, or anhedonia)
B. During the course of the disturbance, functioning in one or more areas such as work, social relations, and self-care has deteriorated markedly from premorbid levels (in the case of a child or adolescent, failure to reach expected level of social or academic development).
C. Signs of the disorder must be present for at least six months.
D. Schizoaffective and mood disorders with psychotic features must be ruled out.
E. The disturbance is not substance-induced or caused by organic factors.
                                                                                      (Sue, Sue & Sue, 1997)

Subtypes of schizophrenia, as mentioned earlier also have specific criteria on the DSM-IV-TR, the criteria for paranoid schizophrenia, disorganized schizophrenia, catatonic schizophrenia and residual schizophrenia can be viewed in Appendix A through D.

Once a diagnosis has been confirmed, the process of therapy and medicating may ensue. These components will be discussed later in this paper.

14

7. Other Conditions (Schizophrenia-like)

The diagnostic criteria for schizophrenia are very detailed to ensure that other medical conditions are not causing the symptoms. There are a number of medical conditions that produce symptoms such as psychosis that may be confused with schizophrenia without a careful examination of the patient. Three of these conditions include bipolar disorder, psychosis and Alzheimer's. Each will be briefly discussed hereafter.

7.1 Bipolar Disorder

This is a fairly common mental illness that used to be referred to as manic depression or manic-depressive disorder. The two distinct poles of this disorder are depression and mania. The confusion occurs as the disorder creates psychotic symptoms such as hallucinations and delusions that could easily be mistaken for symptoms of schizophrenia. The distinguishing factor here is the prominent existence of either mania or depression.

A patient with bipolar disorder, when they are depressed may lack energy and be joyless, sad and uninterested in their world. The despair experienced during this depressed phase can lead to anxiety, restlessness, tension and delusions.

Abnormal excitement, irrational enthusiasm, talkativeness, distractibility, impatience and irritability are all symptoms found in the patient during the manic phase of bipolar disorder. They will tend to have a poor concentration span and have difficulty focusing on one mental idea at a time. Mania manifests in excessive spending, unrealistic goals and an almost unending amount of energy.

The two poles of bipolar disorder may alternate in a rather timely cyclical manner; this cycling can occur in a short period of time or be a slower process. The patient may have a combination of both phases at the same time or one may be fairly constant and dominant over the other. Which ever form is evident in the patient; psychotic symptoms are evident and include delusions and hallucinations (Haycock, 2009).

7.2 Psychosis

Chemical substances have the ability to create psychosis; these substances can range from over-the-counter medications to prescription medications and illegal drugs. It is clear that individuals with a predisposition to psychosis or a history of psychosis are more at risk for the psychosis induced side effects of these drugs.

Steroids and levodopa are prescription medications that increase the levels of dopamine in the brain, with patients with schizophrenia being more susceptible to this side-effect than others. Alcohol and nicotine are legal drugs and the majority of people with schizophrenia are smokers (National Institute of Mental Health). Nicotine stimulates alpha-7 receptors in the brain which creates a soothing effect for the schizophrenic. In contrast however, the nicotine decreases the effect of prescription medication and can

15

result in higher doses of antipsychotic drugs being necessary. Alcohol can cause hallucinations particularly after a binge drinking session, and delusions in conjunction with hallucinations are common when alcohol is withheld from the patient (Haycock, 2009).

Street drugs or illegal drugs often cause psychotic behaviour and should be avoided but particularly by people with schizophrenia. Illegal drugs are often used by patients as a method of escape from their circumstances and as such they will often stop taking their prescription medication which increases the severity of symptoms.

7.3 Alzheimer's Disease

Alzheimer's disease is the most common form of dementia. Alzheimer's is evident in a gradual decline in memory and intellectual ability. Alzheimer's begins with the development of plaque-like material in the brain, tangles of cellular proteins and death of neurons in the cerebral cortex (controls higher order functioning). This decay causes trouble in performing familiar tasks, learning new things, paying attention and understanding events.

Patients with Alzheimer's show psychotic symptoms and may develop paranoia, delusions, hallucinations and behavioural changes. These symptoms are admittedly similar to those of schizophrenia but they develop gradually over several months with a clear loss of short-term memory.

Hardening of arteries in the brain can also cause dementia (cerebral arteriosclerosis) and repeated mini-strokes can damage brain regions from lack of blood supply. This damage can cause psychotic-like symptoms.

Huntington disease is another neurological condition that can be confused with schizophrenia. Huntington's is characterized by mental deterioration and psychotic behaviour (Haycock, 2009).

8. Medication and Schizophrenia

An excess of dopamine in the brain has been implicated in the development of schizophrenia (Cooper, Bloom & Roth, 1986). Antipsychotic drugs have been found to have beneficial effects on schizophrenia by altering the activity of neurotransmitters in the brain. These antipsychotics or neuroleptics help to reduce hallucinations, delusions, bizarre behaviour, aggressive behaviour and thought disorders; they are however less effective in reducing the negative symptoms of schizophrenia. Statistics indicate a 70% reduction in the positive symptoms of schizophrenia in patients using antipsychotics.

Antipsychotic medications are divided into two main categories; first-generation and second-generation (atypical) antipsychotics. First generation medications were introduced in 1954 with chlorpromazine (Thorazine) and were used up to 1990 when clozapine

(Clozaril) was introduced into the market. First-generation antipsychotics include the following:

Brand Name	Generic Name
Haldol	Haloperidol
Loxitane	Loxapine
Mellaril	Thioridazine
Moban	Molindone
Navane	Thiothixene
Orap	Pimozide
Serentil	Mesoridazine
Thorazine	Chlorpromazine
Trilafon	Perphenazine
Prolixin	Fluphenazine
Stelazine	Trifluoperazine
Taractan	Chlorprothixene
Vesprin	Triflupromazine

(Medications for Mental Illness, The Essential Guide to Psychiatric Drugs)
There are unfortunately marked side-effects associated with first-generation medications; these include stiffness, tremors, dry mouth, and weight gain, and sedation, loss of motivation, dizziness and constipation. Even with these side-effects, up to 60% of patients who were treated for a period of six weeks, improved to the point of complete remission.

Atypical antipsychotic medication was introduced into the market in the 1990s. Initially the atypical antipsychotics were marketed as side-effect free, but eventually the side-effects became evident to users. Side effects include insomnia, weight gain, sedation, headaches, constipation and agitation. The second-generation antipsychotics block dopamine in the area of the brain that is associated with psychosis but do not affect the areas responsible for movement coordination. As such, this class of medications produces fewer side-effects than first-generation antipsychotics. The most common second-generation antipsychotics are given in tabular form.

Brand Name	Generic Name
Abilify	Ariiprazole
Clozaril	Clozapine
Geodon	Ziprasidone
Invega	Paliperidone
Risperdal	Risperidone
Seroquel	Quetiapine
Zyprexa	Olanzapine

(Medications for Mental Illness, The Essential Guide to Psychiatric Drugs)

Doctors usually prescribe anti-anxiety medication or minor tranquilizers, such as Ativan, Xanax, Klonopin or Valium when antipsychotic medication is started to reduce the agitation in the patient. In conjunction with antipsychotics, Cogentin or Artane are prescribed to reduce the associated side-effects of the medications.

It is important to acknowledge that many patients will stop taking their medication because of the unpleasant side-effects (Gur & Johnson, 2006).

9. Therapy and Schizophrenia

Prior to the 1950s, psychologists really had little means of controlling the hallucinations and delusions of patients with schizophrenia; this made the concepts of therapy very difficult to carry out. With the advent of antipsychotic medications which lessen the psychotic symptoms of the patient, it became easier for the therapist to engage with the client and thus begin efficacious therapy.

In light of the fact that up to 40% of patients with schizophrenia do not fully overcome their symptoms with a course of medication alone, therapy is an integral part of treatment for the patient with schizophrenia (Gur & Johnson, 2006). It is agreed that a combination of somatic and nonsomatic therapies will produce better results than either alone.

There are a number of approaches used in therapy for patients with schizophrenia, five of which are briefly outlined below:

Supportive Psychotherapy – the basic tenet of this approach is to restore and strengthen the patient's emotional stability and to develop healthy ways of solving problems. This corrective form of therapy combined with medication would be effective in treating schizophrenia. It has also found significant value in treating depression.

Behaviour Therapy – the focus here is to address the undesirable or offensive behaviour. Psychologists will identify the behaviour that is undesirable and work at allowing the patient to 're-learn' more appropriate forms of behaviour. The underlying premise here is that all behaviour is learned and can thus be modified with re-learning.

Cognitive Therapy – this form of therapy focuses attention on the thought-patterns of the patient. It is a relatively short-term therapy that focuses in on specific problems and aims to re-work the 'thoughts' of the patient. Although this form of therapy is not specifically used for patients with schizophrenia, it has been found to be advantageous in working with patients suffering with depression.

Group Therapy – this form of therapy is particularly valuable when working with adolescents. A group of individuals with similar diseases address the issues in a group session. Adolescents are usually more prone to interacting with group members, but as a warning only, this therapy may not be desirable for the more shy, gentle or fragile adolescent.

Family Therapy – this method of therapy is exactly as it suggests. The entire family meets for counseling with the therapist. Adolescent schizophrenia may be triggered by dysfunctional family circumstances and this form of therapy is the perfect opportunity to teach the individuals more appropriate ways of interacting with each other (psycho education).

Schizophrenia involves both biological and physiological factors making a combination of drugs with psychotherapy the most effective approach. The underlying emphasis of therapy should be on social skills training and changing communication patterns among patients and family members (Sue, Sue & Sue, 1997).

10. Hospitalization as an Option

A combination of medication and therapy is effective in the treatment of schizophrenia but the majority of patients with acute schizophrenia will need to be hospitalized. In the case of adolescents, hospitalization is an option if the symptoms become severe.

The reason or purpose of hospitalization is to firstly, correctly diagnose the adolescent and stabilize his medication. Secondly, if the symptoms are severe, the family members, others or the child himself may be at risk of harm. If the child is suicidal or homicidal then hospitalization is a real option. Thirdly, if the adolescent is unable to take care of himself because his behaviour is bizarre or disorganized, then these basic needs can be supplied by the hospital.

The idea of hospitalizing an adolescent is particularly daunting for the parent, but they can take solace in the fact that the majority of treatment that the child will receive for his schizophrenia will take place in outpatient facilities.

11. Conclusion

During the course of this paper we have looked at where schizophrenia began and how its treatment (as barbaric as it seemed) developed. We focused in on the plethora of causes of schizophrenia and realized that there is undoubtedly no single causal factor for this disease but a combination of brain abnormality, genetics and environment that interact in the development of the disease.

We isolated the five different types of schizophrenia and looked their individual characteristics, giving us an understanding of the difficulty in diagnosing schizophrenia. In addition, the positive and negative symptoms of the disease were highlighted and the prevalence discrepancies of males and females, along with suicidal tendencies in schizophrenics were covered.

The focus is adolescent schizophrenia and as such, early warning signs are important because effective management of the disease depends on early identification. The move towards atypical antipsychotic medication was discussed with possible side effects and the combination of pharmacology and therapy was identified as the most effective method of treatment for schizophrenia. In conclusion, we acknowledged the possibility of hospitalization in acute cases and the purpose of hospitalization for the schizophrenic.

12. Appendices – Barlow & Durand (2005)

12.1 Appendix A: DSM-IV-TR Diagnostic Criteria for Paranoid Type

A type of Schizophrenia in which the following criteria are met.

A. Preoccupation with one or more delusions or frequent auditory hallucinations.
B. None of the following is prominent: disorganized speech, disorganized or catatonic behaviour, or flat or inappropriate affect.

12.2 Appendix B: DSM-IV-TR Diagnostic Criteria for Disorganized Type

A type of Schizophrenia in which the following criteria are met.

A. All the following are prominent:
   a. Disorganized speech
   b. Disorganized behaviour
   c. Flat or inappropriate affect
B. The criteria are not met for Catatonic Type.

12.3 Appendix C: DSM-IV-TR Diagnostic Criteria for Catatonic Type

A type of Schizophrenia in which the clinical picture is dominated by at least two of the following:

a. Motoric immobility as evidenced by catalepsy (including waxy flexibility) or stupor
b. Excessive motor activity (that is apparently purposeless and not influenced by external stimuli)
c. Extreme negativism (an apparently motiveless resistance to all instructions or maintenance of a rigid posture against attempts to be moved) or mutism
d. Peculiarities of voluntary movement as evidenced by posturing (voluntary assumption of inappropriate or bizarre postures), stereotyped movements, prominent mannerisms, or prominent grimacing
e. Echolalia or achopraxia

12.4 Appendix D: DSM-IV-TR Diagnostic Criteria for Residual Type

A type of Schizophrenia in which the following criteria are met:

A. Absence of prominent delusions, hallucinations, disorganized speech, and grossly disorganized or catatonic behaviour.
B. There is continuing evidence of the disturbance, as indicated by the presence of negative symptoms or to or more symptoms listed in Criterion A for Schizophrenia, present in an attenuated form (e.g., odd beliefs, unusual perceptual experiences).

13. References

1. Banich, M.T. (2004). *Cognitive Neuroscience and Neuropsychology*. Boston: Houghton Mifflin Company.
2. Barlow, D.H., & Durand, V.M. (2005). *Abnormal Psychology an Integrative Approach*. USA: Wadsworth.
3. Bateson, G., Jackson, D., Haley, J., & Weakland, J. (1956). Toward a theory of schizophrenia. *Behavioural Science, 1,* 251-164.
4. Berk, L.E. (2000). *Child Development 5th Ed.* Massachusetts: Allyn & Bacon.
5. Buchsbaum, M.S. (1990). The frontal lobes, basal ganglia, and the temporal lobes as sites for schizophrenia. *Schizophrenia Bulletin, 16,* 379-389.
6. Castle, D.J., & Murray, R.M. (1993). The epidemiology of late-onset schizophrenia. *Schizophrenia Bulletin, 22,* 691-699.
7. Cooper, J.R., Bloom, F.E., & Roth, R.H. (1986). *The biochemical basis of neuropharmacology (5th ed.).* New York: Oxford University Press.
8. Furnham, A. (2008). *50 Psychology Ideas You Really Need to Know*. London: Quecus Publishing Plc.
9. Gur, R.E., & Johnson, A.B. (2006). *If Your Adolescent has Schizophrenia*. New York: Oxford University Press.
10. Haycock, D.A. (2009). *The Everything Health Guide to Schizophrenia*. Massachusetts: Adams Media.
11. Lieberman, J.A. (1995). Signs and symptoms. *Archives of General Psychiatry, 52,* 361-363.
12. Loehlin, J.C., Willerman, L., & Horn, J.M. (1988). Human behaviour genetics. *Annual Review of Psychology, 38,* 101-133.
13. Reber, A.S., & Reber, E.S. (2001). *The Penguin Dictionary of Psychology*. South Africa: Penguin Books.
14. Sue, D., Sue, D., & Sue, S. (1997). *Understanding Abnormal Behavior*. Boston: Houghton Mifflin Company.
15. Szymanski, S., Kane, J.M., & Lieberman, J.A. (1991). A selective review of biological markers in schizophrenia. *Schizophrenia Bulletin, 17,* 99-111.